DASH Diet for Beginners

Quick and Easy Steps to Lose Weight in 14 Days with DASH Diet (includes Delicious and Irresistible DASH Diet Recipes)

Emma Fisher

Emma Fisher

Copyright © 2015 by Emma Fisher

Legal & Disclaimer

Legal & Disclaimer

The information contained in this book is not designed to replace or take the place of any form of medicine or professional medical advice. The information in this book has been provided for educational and entertainment purposes only.

The information contained in this book has been compiled from sources deemed reliable, and it is accurate to the best of the Author's knowledge; however, the Author cannot guarantee its accuracy and validity and cannot be held liable for any errors or omissions. Changes are periodically made to this book. You must consult your doctor or get professional medical advice before using any of the suggested remedies, techniques, or information in this book.

Upon using the information contained in this book, you agree to hold harmless the Author from and against any damages, costs, and expenses, including any legal fees potentially resulting from the application of any of the information provided by this guide. This disclaimer applies to any damages or injury caused by the use and application, whether directly or indirectly, of any advice or

ii

information presented, whether for breach of contract, tort, negligence, personal injury, criminal intent, or under any other cause of action.

You agree to accept all risks of using the information presented inside this book. You need to consult a professional medical practitioner in order to ensure you are both able and healthy enough to participate in this program.

Emma Fisher

Table of Contents

Introduction

Everyone wants to live a healthy lifestyle. The majority of people, especially during the first few months of a new year make resolutions about making healthier food choices and losing weight. Unfortunately, not everyone is able to stand by their promises; a lot of people actually struggle with fulfilling their diet-related New Year's resolutions just a few weeks after making them. Luckily, you don't need to wait for New Year's Eve to improve your health and make healthier food choices. If you want to prevent yourself from developing all sorts of diseases, or if you want to significantly lower your blood pressure and eventually stop hypertension, then this book is for you.

This book is all about the DASH diet—what it is and how you can try it for yourself. "DASH" simply means Dietary Approach to Stop Hypertension, which as the name denote, a diet that is designed to naturally and effectively boosts your body's nutrients to lower blood pressure. By reading this book, you'll have an idea as to what this diet is all about and how you can start practicing it today. It also contains a lot of diet plans and recipes to help you through this new and healthier way of living. I hope that by the end of reading this book, you would be able to apply all and tips and strategies needed to successfully undergo a DASH diet and reap all the benefits it provides!

Chapter 1: The Rising Cases of Overweight and Obesity

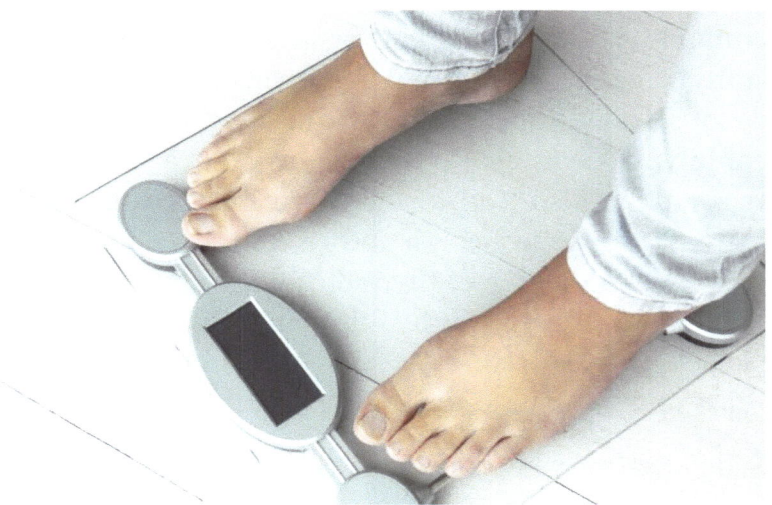

According to the latest statistics of the World Health Organization, 1.9 billion adults all over the world overweight. In this number, 600 million adults are reported to be obese.

Obesity is a condition in which a person has an abnormally high and unhealthy proportion of body fat; it is generally caused by too much eating and lesser physical activities. Consuming high amounts of energy from your diet mostly from fat and sugars, but do not burn off the energy through exercise and physical activity; the excess energy will be stored as body fat.

The balance between calorie intake and energy used up determines a person's weight. When a person consumes more calories than he usually burns, he will gain weight, but if a person eats fewer calories than he usually burns, he will lose weight. Therefore the most common causes of obesity are overeating and physical inactivity.

Obesity may lead to high blood pressure or most commonly known as hypertension. This condition can silently damage your body for years before symptoms develop. If left uncontrolled, you may end up with a disability, a poor quality of life or even a deadly heart attack. It can also lead to increased risk of cancer of the pancreas, esophagus, colon and rectum, breast for women after menopausal stage, thyroid, kidney and gall bladder. Fortunately, with proper health management and lifestyle changes, you can control your high blood pressure to reduce your risk of life-threatening complications.

Besides hypertension, diabetes is another health problem you need to worry about if you do not do anything about your diet. According to The New York Times, the global statistics of diabetes has risen by nearly half over the past two decades. The prevalence of diabetes has been rising not only in rich but in poor countries as well.

While thinking of these diseases may leave you in fear, you do not have to fret because a revolutionary diet is just the answer to that—the Dietary Approaches to Stop Hypertension or what is commonly known as the DASH Diet. This diet was introduced by the National Institute of Health together with different organizations and other related fields across the United States. This diet was created in order to reverse the causes of hypertension and to also help individuals to lose weight and be over-all healthy. Turn to the next chapter to learn more of this diet!

Chapter 2: All About the DASH Diet

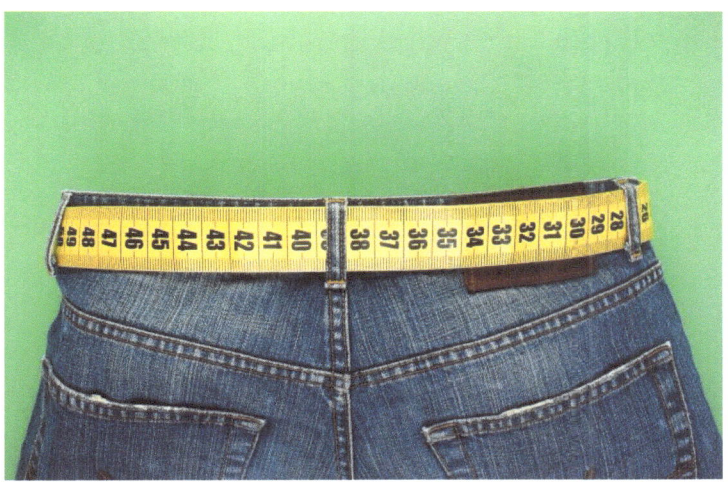

The History of DASH Diet

Due to the rising cases overweight and obesity and other related diseases, the National Institute of Health together with other organizations across the United Sates conducted a comprehensive research on these threatening diseases. The outcome showed that the eating habits of individuals affect their weight which therefore leading them to develop hypertensions. Because of this situation, the DASH Diet or Dietary Approaches to Stop Hypertension was formulated. The DASH Diet intends to lower the blood pressure without any aid of medication; it is an all-natural plan became an established model of healthy eating plan.

How does the DASH Diet work?

The food plan focuses on fruits, vegetables, non-fat/low-fat dairy and whole grains such as cereals. The eating plan also includes the consumption of high fiber foods, medium to low fat diet, low red meat, and less sugar. An additional benefit of this diet is that it is rich in different vitamins and minerals that are important in achieving a healthy body.

Another good thing about this diet plan is that it lowers your sodium intake in your diet (daily consumption for sodium is only 2,300) that will help regulate blood pressure levels. That's because studies show that eating food with high sodium content could lead to a spike in blood pressure.

The diet plan has attested to lower the blood pressure in just two weeks and has been recommended by Centers for Disease Control, American Heart Association, The National Heart, Lung, and Blood Institute, the Mayo Clinic, US guidelines for treatment of high blood pressure and a lot more.

The DASH Diet for Weight Loss

The primary goal of the diet is not actually for weight loss, but with the demand for an effective diet plan that can also solve different health problems, a new DASH Diet research has been conducted to further optimize the present diet plan. Carbs that are not nutritionally balanced were eliminated and more protein-rich food and heart healthy fats were added in the diet, resulting to an effective weight loss diet plan. There are two phases in the diet. Phase One is for the first 14 days of the diet, while Phase Two comes in after 2 weeks in the diet.

Phase 1: Shed Weight Two Weeks

During these 14 days you will learn how to satisfy your hunger with DASH Diet approved foods and as a result, you will feel fuller for a longer time. While whole grains, starchy veggies and fruits are included in the DASH Diet, it's advised that you eliminate these food groups first in the first two weeks of the diet; doing this will help regulate your blood sugar levels and will also curb your cravings for food. Milk is should also be avoided, but you can however, get at least moderated servings of non-fat yogurt.

Amp up your consumption of green veggies such as spinach or other vegetables like broccoli, or cabbage, as well as other vegetables such as cucumbers, peppers and tomatoes.

You can also enjoy up to six ounces of lean meats, fish and poultry a day. Aim for four to five servings of beans or lentils a week.

Be wise in choosing your sources of fat. The best way to get this is by eating fish rich in healthy fats such as salmon and mackerel, or by using oils such as almond oil, olive oil, and almond oil. Absolutely avoid foods that contains saturated and trans fats such as whole-fat dairy, fried foods, vegetable shortening, and store-bought pastries,

Phase 2: Kick It Up a Notch!

After the first 14 days, you will continue eating the foods from Phase 1 but you may start eating some other healthy foods that will help you continue your weight loss. You any choose the following food groups:

Whole Grains: Choose from breads and pasta, cereals, or any items made with whole grain. And totally eliminate foods made from refined grains such as white bread and pasta because these foods cause your blood sugar levels to spike. You can have six to eight servings of whole grains a day.

Fruit: Either fresh or frozen, you should aim to consume four to five servings of fruits daily.

Low-Fat Milk or Yogurt: These are great sources of calcium and Vitamin D. for your body in order to give you strong muscles and bones and also keep your metabolism working.

Sugar-Sugar and other sweets are now allowed in this phase as long as you limit it to not more than five servings a day.

Alcohol- alcohol in the form of wine is allowed in phase two as long as you limit it to a small glass occasionally.

If you really want to live and healthy for the rest of your life, I suggest the you follow the meal plan in phase two and you'll see that you'll be reaping the benefits of DASH Diet in no time.

Benefits of the DASH Diet

Aside from the lowered blood pressure and effective weight loss treatment, several studies also verify that it can prevent other diseases such as cancer, stroke, heart failure, diabetes, kidney stones, and osteoporosis.

For diabetes, the high-fiber food consumption of DASH Diet (minimum intake is about 30g of fiber daily) does not only help promote a better digestion, but it can also control glucose and insulin production; which also makes a great food plan for diabetics.

The other advantages of DASH diet are: reverse ageing effects, strengthen the bones, joints and muscles, rejuvenate the hair and skin, reduce cholesterol level, cut risk factor of metabolic syndrome, and improve heart health. Exercise or regular workouts are recommended with the DASH Diet in order to reap further health benefits.

Remember, this diet is not just any fad diet, or once you achieved your health/weight goals in an "x" amount of time, you will quit the diet. The point of the diet is an overall lifestyle change to be maintained for a healthier you.

Chapter 3: The DASH Diet Menu

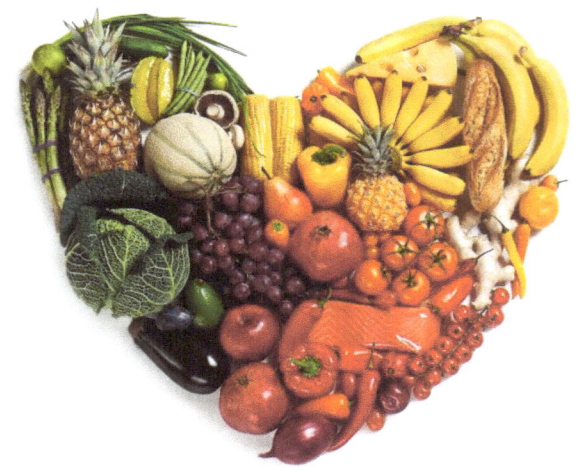

These are the following foods that make up a DASH Diet Menu:

Vegetables—eat plenty of vegetables! Veggies are not only a great source of fiber that enables good digestion, but they are rich in vitamins and minerals that are essential to a healthy body. Choose from asparagus, beets, bell peppers, broccoli, cabbage, carrots, cauliflower, celery, corn, cucumbers, eggplant, green beans, jicama, mushrooms and leafy greens such as kale, lettuce, and spinach. You should however, limit your consumption of starchy vegetables especially during the first phase of the diet.

Whole Grains—like granola, whole grain bead, and oats. (Do not mistake whole grains with mixed grains because they are two different things.)

Fruits—avocados, apples, bananas, berries, grapefruit, grapes, lemon and lime, cantaloupe, peaches, etc. are also included in the DASH Diet list. You can consume fruits either fresh or by making smoothies out of them. Just remember to stick to the recommended servings a day.

Meat, Poultry, and Seafood—pick organic, grass-fed, or wild caught. Stick to lean meats and deli meats low in sodium. Eggs are also great source of protein, but you could also choose to use egg substitutes instead.

Herbs & Spices (dried or fresh)—skip the salt and flavor your foods with herbs and spices such as basil, oregano, thyme, rosemary, dill, bay leaf, curry, coriander, cayenne pepper, chilies, cumin, chives, parsley, garlic, onions, ginger, mint, mustard, paprika, etc.

Nuts and Seeds—choose the unsalted or raw variety of almonds, cashews, hazelnuts, sunflower seeds, and pumpkin seeds.

Beverages—Avoid sugar-laden beverages such as soda and artificially flavored juices and stick to 100% fruit juice, tea, vegetable juice, and most especially, water.

Here are the foods that you should avoid:

Food high rich sugar or Fructose— this has been considered unhealthy because it provides empty calories. Refined sugar has a lot of calories but NO essential nutrients.

Trans fats—also known as "hydrogenated" or "partially hydrogenated" fats. These are unsaturated fats that have been chemically modified to increase food's shelf-life and make them solid at room temperature.

Dairy Products—derive from animals can also introduce additional saturated fat into your diet. These foods include: creams, cheeses, milk, sour cream, ice cream.

Fats and Oils—high saturated fat foods that are in this category include: butter, lard, and certain oils such as palm oil, cream based dressings or dips.

Chapter 4: DASH Diet Meal Portions

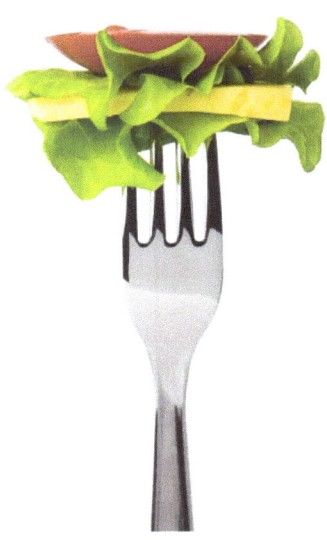

As a daily –suggested serving you must consume at least 2,000 calories per day.

Vegetables—consume four to five servings of vegetables a day. You can make veggies sticks as snacks other being served as a side dish in order to reach the recommended daily consumption. The more veggies you munch on, the better.

Fruits—four to five daily servings of fruit daily are also recommended in the DASH Diet. One serving is equal to a medium fruit or half a cup of freshly squeezed (100%) fruit.

Grains—is a good source of energy and fiber, whole-grains should be eaten up at least six to eight servings a day. A piece of whole-wheat bread is an example of one serving. You may also want to add grains such as oats, pita bread, brown rice, and whole-grain pasta in your diet.

Dairy—is a good source of calcium and protein in this diet. Two to three servings of this is suggested for this diet. One cup of low-fat yogurt is a good example of a single serving.

Fish, Poultry and Meat- as a source of protein you can have not more than six servings a day of fish and or Poultry and Meat. Eat only the lean parts, you must also remove the skin of the chicken and it is best cook by broiling, or grilling. Eggs are allowed in this diet but eat only four eggs a week because of the high cholesterol content found in the egg yolks,.

Sweets—sweets is also allowed in the DASH Diet but you have to keep it to a maximum of five servings per week.

Fats, Oils—good sources of fat such as olive oil, avocado, and coconut oil. You can only have two servings per day.

Nuts, Seeds, and Legumes—the only five servings per week of these are allowed per week.

DASH Diet has many food choices that would make delicious meals that are easy to prepare. But you should keep in mind that moderation is still the key to this diet to get good results in just a short period of time.

Chapter 5: The Dos and Don'ts of the DASH Diet

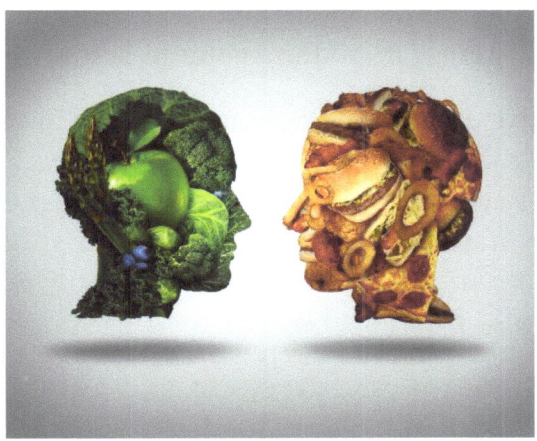

Remember these Dos and Don'ts so you would benefit from the DASH diet:

Do'

Be wise in choosing your food. The flexibility of this diet is so simple that you can eat almost anything in moderation.

Satisfy your sweet tooth with fruits. Instead of eating chocolates and candies to satisfy your sweet cravings you may opt to eat fruits and other DASH recipes that is easy to prepare. All you need is determination and discipline.

Choose what you eat. Food manufacturers nowadays have already addressed the needs of the health conscious customers. They offer an array of food selections that you can choose from. Almost all of them have a DASH-friendly product for you.

Like, if you need to buy dairy products, you choose the low-fat or non-fat products. Buy the unrefined sugar instead of getting the refined white sugar. But, if you have no option but to buy canned goods, be sure to rinse its sodium content before coking.

Enjoy cooking. Cooking your own food is the best and safest way to maintain your diet. This lessens the risk that you may be eating too much of your daily nutritional intakes if you order your food from restaurants. Learning to cook not only is safer but it can also be enjoyable.

Eat lean poultry, meat and fish in moderation. These food are good for the heart and is a healthy choice, they are low-fat diet

Go for whole grains and vegetables. Many of the whole grain foods are rich in fiber, calcium, protein and potassium, which have been revealed to help fend off or lower high blood pressure.

Don'ts

Begin without preparation. Compared to other diets offered, DASH diet is relatively easy but to make it more effective, you must it preparation yourself before starting it. Begin by weighing yourself first so you can monitor your progress. Prepare yourself by making sure you will follow the diet strictly and make it habit and a lifestyle. Next is to prepare your grocery list making sure you have the DASH- friendly food groups to meet your nutritional intake.

Replace the diet for your medication. This diet is meant to supplement not replace any current medications you are taking. This is not an all-in-one solution; if you are on a prescribed medication, DASH Diet is one of the best healthy meals plans out there. To be safe, get a green light from your doctor first before starting the diet, especially if you already have an existing condition.

Take too much salt. Seasoning your dishes herbs, spices or lemon zest is the best way to benefit from DASH diet. Salt makes your food taste delicious, but it should be used in moderate amounts. Consuming more sodium than the maximum recommended daily intake is harmful. This can cause diseases such as hypertension, edema or too much fluid retention in the body, hypernatremia or levels of sodium in your body are higher than is normal, and cardiovascular disease.

Starting the diet sooner, the more benefits you can gain. DASH Diet needs a moderately small amount of preparation and no substantial changes are needed in your food choices. Begin now and gain your desired weight soon!

Chapter 6: DASH Diet Recipes

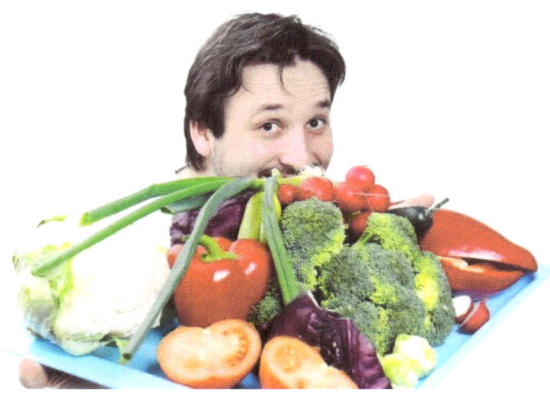

Here are some DASH Diet Recipes for breakfast, lunch, and dinner.

DASH Diet Recipes for Breakfast

#1 Cauliflower and Cheese Omelets

(Serves 4)

Ingredients:

4 cups cauliflower cut into small parts
4 eggs (preferably organic)
2 egg whites
½ cup parmesan cheese, shredded
1 tbsp. light olive oil
salt and pepper to taste

Preparation:

1. Set oven at 350°F.

2. Place cauliflower in the steamer and cook for about six minutes or until tender.

3. Transfer steamed cauliflower into a bowl and mash into smaller pieces. Drizzle with olive oil and season with salt and pepper. Combine well.

4. Spray a muffin pan with cooking spray and pour the mixture into the tins.

5. In another bowl, whisk the whole eggs, whites and grated parmesan cheese. Mix well.

6. Pour the egg mixture into the tins over cauliflower filling up to ¾ for the tin.

7. Place in the oven and cook for at least twenty minutes.

8. Serve immediately.

Serve this omelet with a fruit salad, whole-wheat toast, and a glass of low-fat milk and enjoy a complete well-balanced and delicious breakfast.

Nutrition Information:

Serving Size: 1 mini-omelet
Per Serving: 104 calories, 7 g total fat, 3 g of carbohydrates

#2 Peanut Butter & Banana Breakfast Smoothie

(Serves 1)

Ingredients:

1 8 oz. non-fat milk
1 tablespoon all natural peanut butter
1 medium banana, frozen or fresh

Preparation:

1. Combine all ingredients in blender, and mix until very smooth.

Nutrition Information:

Per serving: 285 calories, 8.4 g total fat, 1 g saturated fat, 42 g carbohydrates, 13 g protein, 4 g fiber, 186 mg sodium, 882 mg potassium, 32 mg magnesium, 506 mg calcium

#3 Monkey Pancakes

(Serves 6)

Ingredients:

1 cup whole-wheat flour
2 tsp. baking powder

1/8 tsp. kosher salt

¼ tsp. cinnamon powder

1 cup almond milk
1 ripe banana, mashed
3 egg whites

2 tsp. canola oil
1 tsp. vanilla extract
2 tbsp. walnuts, chopped

1 tsp. almond oil

Preparation:

1. Place all the dry ingredients in a bowl and mix well.
2. In a separate bowl, whisk the almond milk, canola oil, egg whites and vanilla extract. Add the mashed bananas and combine well.
3. Gradually add the dry ingredients into the wet ingredients and mix well using a spatula until all are totally mixed.
4. Place a non-stick pan coated with a small amount of almond oil over medium fire.
5. Pour ¼ cup batter into the pan and cook until bubble starts to appear. Flip the pancake and cook for another 2-3 minutes.
6. Repeat with the remainder of the batter.

Omit the syrup instead top it with one cup of non-fat vanilla   yogurt.

Nutrition Information:

Per serving: 146 calories, 4 g total fat, 1 g saturated fat, 22 g carbohydrates, 7 g protein, 3 g fiber, 331 mg sodium, 201 mg potassium, 39 mg magnesium, 95 mg calcium

#4 Eggs and Tomato Breakfast Melts
(Serves 4)

Ingredients:

2 whole-grain English Muffins, cut in half
1 tsp. light olive oil
8 egg whites, beaten
4 finely chopped leeks

salt and black pepper, to taste

½ cup shredded reduced-fat Swiss cheese

½ cup cherry tomatoes, cut in half

Preparation:

1. Preheat the griller on high. Place muffins, cut side up, and grill for 2 minutes or until the edges are beginning to turn light brown. (In case a griller is not available you can also use an oven toaster.)

2. Heat a pan on medium heat. Add oil and sauté three pcs. of leeks for about 2 to 3 minutes. Add the egg whites, season with salt and pepper and cook, mixing it with a wooden spoon until cooked.

3. Divide on toasted muffins and top with tomatoes, cheese and remaining leeks.

4. Grill for 1 to 1 1/2 minutes or until cheese has melted, careful not to burn.

Nutrition Information:

Per serving: Calories 162; Total Fat 6 g; Saturated Fat 3 g; Carbohydrates 16 g; Protein 13 g; Fiber 3 g; Sodium 283 mg (without salt); Potassium 235 mg; Magnesium 38 mg; Calcium 204 mg

#5 Fruit Pizza
(Serves 2)

Ingredients:

1 English muffin (choose whole-grain)

2 tbsp. fat-free cream cheese

2 tbsp. sliced strawberries

2 tbsp. blueberries

¼ part of an apple, cut into cubes
2 tbsp. crushed pineapple

Preparation:

1. Cut the English muffin into two and toast the halves until lightly browned.

2. Spread cream cheese on both halves.

3. Equally divide the fruits between the two muffin halves, arranging them on top of cream cheese.

4. Serve   while   it   is   hot.

(A good substitute of cream cheese is peanut butter or yogurt.)

Nutrition Information:

Serving size = one half muffin with fruit. Per serving: 120 calories, 3 g total fat, 1.5 g saturated fat, 19 g carbohydrates, 4 g protein, 3 g fiber, 190 mg sodium, 143 mg potassium, 28 mg magnesium, 114 mg calcium

#6 Almond Rice Pudding

(Serves 6)

Ingredients:

3 cups low-fat milk
1 cup brown rice
¼ cup sugar
1 tsp. vanilla extract
¼ tsp. almond extract
½ tsp. cinnamon powder

¼ cup toasted almonds (optional)

Preparation:

1. In a medium saucepan mix the milk and rice, and bring to a boil.
2. Reduce heat and boil for another thirty minutes with the lid on or until the rice is soft.
3. Remove the saucepan from the fire and then mix the almond and vanilla extract and cinnamon powder.
4. Sprinkle toasted almonds on top and serve warm.
5. Serve together with one tall glass of freshly squeezed orange.

Nutrition Information:

Serving size: ½ cup
Per serving: 180 calories, 1.5 g total fat, 1 g saturated fat, 36 g carbohydrates, 7 g protein, 1 g fiber, 65 mg sodium, 1 mg potassium, 0 mg magnesium, 150 mg calcium

#7 Baked Stuffed Apples
(Serves 4)

Ingredients:

4 large apples
1/4 cup coconut flakes
1/4 cup chopped dried apricots
2 tsp. grated orange zest
1/2 cup orange juice
2 tbsp. brown sugar

Preparation:

1. With a knife, peel the top of the apples and hollow out the center.
2. Combine coconut flakes, apricots, and orange zest; divide to evenly fill centers of apples.
3. Arrange the apples in a microwave-safe baking dish.
4. Mix orange juice and brown sugar and pour over apples.
5. Place in microwave and cook on high heat for 7 to 8 minutes or until apples are tender. Cool before serving. Serve it together with a low- fat milk

Nutrition Information:

Per serving: 192 calories, 2 g total fat, 1 g saturated fat, 46 g carbohydrates, 1 g protein, 6 g fiber, 19 mg sodium, 276 mg potassium, 15 mg magnesium, 22 mg calcium

DASH Diet Recipes For Lunch

#1 Quick and Easy Stir Fry
(Serves: 4)

Ingredients:

1 lb. chicken fillet, cut into cubes

2 cups broccoli florets

1/3 cup freshly squeezed orange juice
1 tbsp. light soy sauce
1 tbsp. *homemade oriental sauce
2 tsp. cornstarch
1 tbsp. light olive oil
1 6-oz frozen snow peas
2 cups red cabbage, shredded

*Ingredients for Oriental Sauce

1 cup water
10 pcs. dried chilies, stems and seeds removed
6 cloves of garlic
salt to taste
1 ½ tsp. cornstarch dissolved in 1 tablespoon of water
2 tbsp. sesame oil
1 clove garlic, finely chopped
1 tsp. ginger, minced
1 tbsp. celery, finely chopped
2 tbsp. spring onions, finely chopped
2 tbsp. ketchup
1 ½ teaspoons white vinegar

Preparation for the Oriental Sauce

1. Pour ½ cup of water in a saucepan, add in chilies, and garlic and simmer for at least eight minutes. Set aside and allow to cool.

2. Put the mixture in a blender to create a smooth paste. Add small amount of water if needed.

3. Then add the remaining ½ cup of water and thin it out.

4. Heat up the pan in a medium fire and add in the minced ginger, garlic, celery and green onion.

5. Mix in prepared chili-garlic mixture and salt. Let it simmer.

6. Add prepared cornstarch mixture and stir.

7. Add in ketchup, and vinegar, mix well.

8. Cook till it gets thick for about 2 minutes, or until the oil floats up.

9. Turn off heat.

10. Scoop 1 tbsp. of the sauce.

11. Pack in a clean container the remaining use for future use.

Preparation for the Stir-Fry:

1. Whisk the orange juice, soy sauce, oriental sauce, and cornstarch in a bowl and set aside.
2. In a pan heat the oil and add chicken. Stir -fry until chicken is cooked (about 5 minutes).
3. Throw in the vegetables and peas and the prepared oriental sauce. Cook for another few minutes or until vegetables are almost done. Do not overcook.
4. Garnish with sesame seeds and serve with brown rice on the side.

Nutrition Information:

Per Serving: 340 Calories, 8g Total Fat, 35g Carbohydrate, 28g Protein, 5g Fiber, 240 mg Sodium, 80 mg Calcium

#2 Bean and Barley Burgers
(Serves 8)

Ingredients:

1/2 tsp. garlic powder
2 cups cooked kidney beans
1/2 cup wheat germ
1 tbsp. olive oil
1/2 cup chopped onion
 3 minced garlic cloves, minced
1 tsp. salt
1/2 tsp. sage
1/2 tsp. ground celery seeds
 2 cups cooked whole barley (hull removed)

Preparation:

1. In a saucepan cook beans and barley until soft, then mash beans and barley together.
2. In a separate pan, fry onion and garlic in oil until golden.
3. Add to bean and barley mixture along with spices and wheat germ and stir to combine.
4. Form into 4" patties and fry on medium heat until brown on both sides.
5. Put burgers on a whole wheat bun with a sliced tomato, lettuce, and avocado.

Serve along with a freshly squeezed lemon juice and salad with vinaigrette dressing.

Nutrition Information:

Per serving: 280 calories, 4 g total fat, 0 g saturated fat, 49 g carbohydrates, 12 g protein, 13 g fiber, 300 mg sodium, 198 mg potassium, 40 mg magnesium

#3 Chicken in Cranberry Sauce

(Serves 4)

Ingredients:

16 oz. chicken breasts, skinned and bones removed
1 tsp. ghee
¼ tsp. pepper
¾ cup whole cranberry sauce
¼ cup chili sauce
¼ cup apple juice
1 tsp. brown sugar

Preparation:

1. Gently pound the chicken and then season with pepper.
2. Heat ghee in a skillet over medium-high fire and cook until chicken turns slightly brown.
3. Add in the rest of the ingredients and let it simmer for at least 15 minutes.
4. Remove the pan cover and boil until the sauce is at desired thickness.

Serve with your favorite steamed vegetables, and glass of chilled low-fat milk to make this DASH meal complete.

Nutrition Information: Serving size ¼ pound Per Serving: 302 calories, 5g total fat, 27g carbohydrates, 35 g protein, 1 g of fiber, 333 mg sodium, 291 mg potassium, 33 mg magnesium, 18 mg calcium.

#4. Quick and Easy Pasta and Broccoli
(Serves 6)

Ingredients:

12 oz. uncooked pasta

7 cups broccoli florets,

5 cloves of smashed and chopped garlic
¼ cup parmesan cheese, grated
2 tbsp. light olive oil, divided
salt and cracked pepper, to taste

Preparation:

1. Place water (about 4-5 cups) in a large pot and bring to a boil.

2. Add in pasta and broccoli at the same time and cook until the pasta is al dente. When the pasta is almost done, set aside 1 cup of water used to cook the pasta.
3. Drain pasta and broccoli.
4. Put the pot back on the stove and heat over medium-high fire.
5. Add 1 tbsp. of oil. Once hot, add garlic until golden then reduce heat to low.
6. Add pasta back to the pot. Mix well.
7. Add remaining olive oil and grated cheese.
8. Mix well and sure to smash any large pieces of broccoli.
9. Add ½ cup of the reserved pasta water and mix well, adding more if needed.
10. Add salt and pepper to taste.

Pair it with freshly squeeze orange juice to complete your nutritious DASH meal.

Nutrition Information:

Per serving (without added salt): 289 calories, 7 g total fat, 1 g saturated fat, 48 g carbohydrates, 12 g protein, 5 g fiber, 104 mg sodium, 346 mg potassium, 52 mg magnesium, 89 mg calcium.

#5. Zesty Chicken Stir Fry

(Serves 4)

Ingredients:

4 pcs. chicken breast, skin removed and cut it into cubes

1/2 cup chicken broth

2 tbsp. light soy sauce

2 tsp. cornstarch

2 tbsp. water

3 tsp. canola or corn oil, divided

1 bunch asparagus, trimmed and cut into 2-inch pieces

6 cloves of chopped garlic

1 tbsp. fresh ginger

3 tbsp. fresh lemon juice

salt and pepper to taste

Preparation:

1. Lightly season the chicken with salt.
2. Mix chicken broth and soy sauce in a small bowl.
3. In another bowl, combine the cornstarch and water and mix well.
4. Heat a non-stick pan over medium-high fire.
5. Add 1 tsp. of oil, then add the asparagus and cook until tender-crisp for about 3 to 4 minutes.
6. Then add the ginger and garlic and then sauté for about 1 minute or until golden. Set aside.
7. Increase the heat to high, then add 1 teaspoon of oil and half of the chicken and cook until browned and cooked well, about 4 minutes on each side.
8. Remove and set aside and repeat with the remaining oil and chicken. Set aside.
9. Add the soy sauce mixture; bring to a boil and cook about 1-1/2 minutes.
10. Add in lemon juice and cornstarch mixture and stir well, when it simmers return the chicken and asparagus to the pan and mix well.

Serve it with chilled apple juice to enjoy your meal.

Nutritional Information:

Per 1 1/4 cups serving: Calories 268 • Fat: 7 g • Carb: 10 g • Fiber: 3 g • Protein: 41 g • Sugar: 0 g Sodium: 437 mg (without salt) • Cholesterol: 98 mg

#6. Peruvian Stir Fried Beef

(Serves 2)

Ingredients:

For the Baked Fries:

cooking spray
1 medium potato
1 tsp. olive oil
1/4 tsp. garlic powder
salt and black pepper, to taste

For the Beef:

1/2 lb. lean sirloin, cut into small, thin strips
salt and black pepper to taste
1/4 tsp. cumin
1 tsp. olive oil
1 medium-sized onion, sliced into thick strips
1 large yellow bell pepper
1 large jalapeno, seeds removed and chopped

2 cloves of garlic, crushed

1 medium tomato, sliced into wedges

1 1/2 tbsp. low sodium soy sauce

1 tbsp. apple cider vinegar

1/4 cup chopped cilantro

Preparation:

1. Preheat oven to 400°F.
2. Lightly coat the baking sheet with cooking spray.
3. Cut the potato lengthwise into 1/3-inch thick fries.
5. Put the potatoes on the baking sheet, drizzle with olive oil and toss evenly to coat.
6. Season with garlic powder, salt and pepper.
7. Bake uncovered in the oven for about 25 minutes or until tender crisp and golden.
8. To prepare the beef, season meat with salt, pepper and cumin.
9. Heat a large pan over high temperature. When the pan is hot, add the oil and the steak and cook about 2 minutes, until browned on both sides.
10. Add the onions, bell pepper, jalapeno and garlic and cook 2 minutes.
11. Add in the tomato, soy sauce and vinegar and cook 1 more minute.
12. Season with more salt as needed, remove from heat and finish with cilantro.
13. Serve immediately with french fries.

Nutritional Information:

1/2 of the recipe : Calories 308.5 • Fat: 9 g • Carb: 28 g • Fiber: 4 g • Protein: 28 g • Sugar: 3 g Sodium: 522 mg (without salt) • Cholesterol: 48 mg

#7. Salad Ama-Zing!

(Serves 4)

Ingredients:

16 oz. cooked jumbo shrimp (skin and vein removed), chopped
1 tomato, diced
1 Haas avocado, diced
1 jalapeno pepper, seeds removed and diced
¼ cup onion, chopped
1 cup of lime juice
1 tsp. olive oil
1 tbsp. fresh cilantro, chopped
salt and pepper to taste

Preparation:

1. Mix the onion, lime juice, olive oil in a bowl and season with salt and pepper. Set aside and let it rest for five minutes.
2. In another bowl, mix together chopped shrimp, tomato, jalapeño and avocado.
3. Drizzle he olive oil and lime juice mixture over the shrimp and toss all the ingredients together. Add the chopped cilantro and toss again.

Nutritional Information:

Serving Size: 7/8 cup • Old Points: 4 pt • Points+: 5 pt Calories: 210.4 • Fat: 9.2 g • Protein: 25.1 g • Carb: 7.8 g • Fiber: 3.6 g • Sugar: 0.6 Sodium without salt: 260.8 mg

DASH Diet Recipes for Dinner

#1 Grilled Salmon

(Serves 4)

Ingredients:

(1 1/4-pound) boneless salmon fillet
1 lemon, halved
3/4 tsp. salt
1 tsp. dried oregano
1/8 tsp. black pepper
a few stems fresh oregano and thyme (optional)
1 cup medium- sized tomatoes, halved
1/4 cup sliced red onion
1/4 cup olives, quartered in long strips
1 tsp. olive oil
1 tsp. red wine vinegar
fresh oregano for garnish

Preparation:

1. Cut 1/2 of the lemon into thin slices.
2. Season fish with the remaining juice from 1/2 lemon, salt, oregano and black pepper .
3. Cover and refrigerate until ready to grill.
4. In a bowl, mix the tomatoes, onion, olives, oil and vinegar. Season with salt and pepper.
5. Heat the grill to medium-high heat.
6. Close the lid and allow the grill get hot.
7. Place salmon on the direct heat and cook for 8 to 10 minutes, depending on the thickness, or until done. Turn it to cook the other side. (Use fork to take a peak if it is done)

8. When the fish is cooked, top with tomato mixture and serve.

Serve it with fresh lemon juice.

Nutritional Information:

Serving Size: 1/4 Calories: 251 • Fat: 11 • Carbs: 8 g • Fiber: 2 • Protein: 30 g • Sugar: 0 g
Sodium: 393 mg • Cholesterol: 78 mg

#2 Veggie Lasagna

(Serves   8)

Ingredients:

2 large zucchini
1 lb. ground beef (preferably grass-fed)
4 cloves of garlic, chopped
1 small onion, chopped
1 tsp. light olive oil
28 oz. can low-sodium crushed tomatoes
2 tbsp. fresh basil, chopped
¼ cup ricotta cheese
¼ cup parmesan cheese
¼ cup mozzarella cheese, shredded
1 egg
salt and pepper to taste

Preparation:

1. Brown the meat in a saucepan over medium-high fire. Transfer into a bowl and drain any excess oil.
2. Using the same pan, sauté garlic and onions with 1 tbsp. of olive oil until the onions caramelize.

3. Place the beef back to the pan then pour crushed tomatoes and basil. Season with salt and pepper. Cover and let it simmer on low fire for about 35-40 minutes.

4. While waiting for the sauce to cook, cut zucchini into thick slices; add a small amount of salt and set aside for 10 minutes.

5. Using a paper towel, blot moisture from zucchini and place on the grill to cook over medium heat for about two minutes on each side.

6. Combine the ricotta and parmesan in a bowl with the egg and stir well.

7. Take an oven-safe dish and spread the tomato and beef and tomato sauce at the bottom.

8. Lay zucchini slices on top and then place some of the cheese mixture on top and repeat the process.

9. Pour sauce on top and cover with shredded mozzarella cheese.

10. Cover with aluminum foil and place in the oven for about 45 minutes at 375°F.

11. Remove the cover and cook again for another 15 minutes.

12. Let it cool before serving.

Nutritional Information

Serving Size: 1/8 Calories: 345 • Fat: 17 g • Carbs: 16 g • Fiber: 2 g • Protein: 36 g • Sugar: 8 g
Sodium: 801 (without salt)

#3 Grilled Chicken with Luscious Salsa

(Serves   4)

Ingredients:

3 medium-sized tomatoes
2 small cloves of garlic, minced
¼ cup onion, onion
2 tbsp. basil leaves, chopped
1 tbsp. light olive oil
1 tbsp. balsamic vinegar
salt and pepper to taste
20 oz. chicken cutlets, thinly sliced

Preparation:

1. Whisk in a bowl the onion, oil, and balsamic vinegar. Season with salt and pepper and set aside.

2. Chop the tomatoes and place in a separate bowl.

3. Add the oil mixture with the tomatoes and another pinch of salt and pepper. Set aside in the fridge.

4. Preheat the grill to medium-high.

5. Grill the chicken (seasoned with salt and pepper) for about two minutes on each side, transfer on a platter and top with the tomato-balsamic chilled salsa.

6. Best eaten with toasted garlic bread.

Nutritional Serving:

Serving Size: 2 cutlets + tomatoes : Calories: 237 • Fat: 8.5 g • Protein: 32 g • Carb: 7 g • Fiber: 1 g • Sugar: 0.5 g Sodium: 182.9 mg (without the salt)

#4 Orange Chicken Twist

(Serves   4)

Ingredients:

For the Orange Sauce:

1/3 cup freshly-squeezed orange juice
1/4 cup chicken broth
2 tbsp. soy sauce
2 tbsp. sugar
1 tbsp. Chinese rice wine
1 tbsp. chili paste or more according to taste
1 tbsp. rice vinegar
1/4 tsp. white pepper
2 tsp. cornstarch

For the chicken:

20 oz. chicken breast, skinless and deboned, cut into small cubes
salt, to taste
1 1/2 tbsp. cornstarch
4 tsp. sesame oil, divided
4 cloves minced garlic
1-inch grated ginger
1 tsp. grated orange zest
2 tbsp. chopped scallions
1/2 tsp. sesame seeds, for garnishing

Preparation:

1. Mix the orange sauce ingredients and set aside.

2. Season the chicken with small amount salt and coat evenly with cornstarch, set aside.

3. Heat the pan on high heat, add 1 teaspoon of sesame oil and add half of the chicken.

4. Cook 2 to 3 minutes on each side until evenly browned; set aside.

5. Add 1 teaspoon of oil and chicken and repeat cooking 2 to 3 minutes on each side. Set aside with the rest of the chicken.

6. Add remaining teaspoon of oil and quickly stir-fry the minced garlic and ginger until fragrant, about 1 minute.

7. Add the orange zest and then return the chicken to the pan.

8. Quickly stir the chicken then add the orange sauce and cook until the sauce thickens, about 1 to 2 minutes.

9. Divide between 4 plates and garnish with scallions and sesame seeds.

10. Enjoy this dish with a freshly squeezed lemon juice.

Nutritional Information:
Size: generous 3/4 cup : Calories: 288 • Fat: 9 g • Carb: 18 g • Fiber: 0.5 g • Protein: 32.5 g • Sugar: 9 g
Sodium: 463 mg • Cholesterol: 81 mg

#5 Healthy Baked Chicken Nuggets

(Serves 4)

Ingredients:
2 large chicken fillets

3 tsp. olive oil, divided
8 tbsp. breadcrumbs
2 tbsp. parmesan cheese, grated
salt and pepper to taste
olive oil for greasing

Preparation:

1. Set oven to 425° F

2. In a bowl, combine breadcrumbs, 1 tbsp. olive oil and cheese.

3. Cut the chicken into bite sized pieces and season it with salt and pepper.

4. Coat the nuggets with the remaining olive oil. And then roll them on the breadcrumbs and cheese mixture.

5. Lay the nuggets on a baking sheet coated with cooking spray and then place in the oven and cook for five minutes. Turn over the nuggets and then cook for another five minutes.

Enjoy it along with your favorite salad.

Nutritional Information:

Serving Size: 1/4th of nuggets: Calories: 164.9 • Fat: 4.6 g • Protein: 22.1 g • Carb: 7.7 g • Fiber: 0.9 g • Sugar: 0.1 g

#6 Double "S" Baked Pasta

(Serves   8)

Ingredients:

¾ lb. chicken sausage
1 ¼ cups baby spinach
½ cup parmesan, grated
½ cup low-fat cheddar, shredded
½ cup mozzarella cheese, shredded
12 oz. rigatoni pasta
2 tsp. olive oil, divided
salt and pepper to taste

4 cups Quick Marinara Sauce*

Ingredients for Quick Marinara Sauce

1 tsp. light olive oil
2 cloves garlic, roughly chopped
28 oz. can crushed tomatoes
2 tbsp. chopped fresh basil
1 tsp. oregano
salt and pepper to taste

Preparation for Marinara:

1. Heat olive oil in a pan over medium fire.

2. Add garlic and sauté for 2-3 minutes or until golden.

3. Throw in the tomatoes, oregano, bay leaf and season with salt and pepper.

4. Stir constantly over low heat.

5. Cover and let simmer for about 15 minutes. Remove from heat and add fresh basil. Set aside.

Preparation for Double "S" Pasta:

1. Preheat the oven to 375°F.

2. Cook pasta according to packaging directions. Drain water in a colander and place back paste in the pot.

3. Remove sausage from its casing and place on a heated skillet. Cook until the sausages turn brown and start to crumble. Set aside.

4. Add 1 tbsp. oil to the skillet and throw in garlic. Cook for one minute before adding the spinach.

5. Place the meat crumbles back to the skillet with the spinach and cook for another 4-5 minutes. Season with salt and pepper.

6. Pour the prepared marinara and sausage and spinach into the pot with the cooked pasta. Mix well.

7. Combine the cheeses in a bowl.

8. Transfer the Double "S" pasta into a large baking dish and cover with cheese mixture on top. Cover the dish with aluminum foil.

9. Place in the oven to cook for about twenty minutes. Remove the cover and cook for

another seven minutes, or until the cheese has melted.

10. Let it cool before serving.

Nutritional Information:

Size: 1 3/4 cups Calories: 398 • Fat: 12.5 g • Protein: 27.5 g • Carbs: 44 g • Fiber: 6 g • Sugar: 1.5 g
Sodium: 636 mg (without salt)

#7 Tilapia in Thai Sauce

(Serves   6)

Ingredients:

6 pcs. of 6-oz. tilapia fillets
1 tsp. sesame oil, divided
1 tbsp. fresh ginger, minced
4 cloves or garlic, minced
1 cup red bell pepper, chopped
1 cup leeks, chopped
1 tsp. curry powder
2 tsp. red curry paste
1/2 tsp. cumin, ground
4 tsp. light soy sauce
1 tbsp. brown sugar
2 tsp. fish sauce
14 oz. can coconut milk
1/4 cup cilantro, chopped
salt to taste
cooking oil

Preparation:

1. Preheat broiler.

2. In a large pan heat ½ tsp. of oil over medium fire.

3. Add in ginger and garlic, pepper, and leeks and cook for about a minute or two.

4. Add the curry powder, paste and ground cumin; cook for another minute.

5. Mix in the soy sauce, fish sauce and sugar.

6. Lastly, add coconut milk and bring to a simmer, but do not boil.

7. Remove from heat and stir in cilantro or basil.

8. Meanwhile, brush fish with the remaining ½ tsp. oil and season with salt.

9. Place fish on a baking sheet coated with a small amount of cooking spray.

10. Broil for about 5-7 minutes or until fish is flaky. Cover with the fish with the coconut sauce before serving.

Nutritional Information:

Serving Size: 1 piece fish plus sauce Calories: 225.2
• Fat: 6.9 g Protein: 35.5 g • Carb: 5.6 g • Fiber: 1.1 g

Conclusion

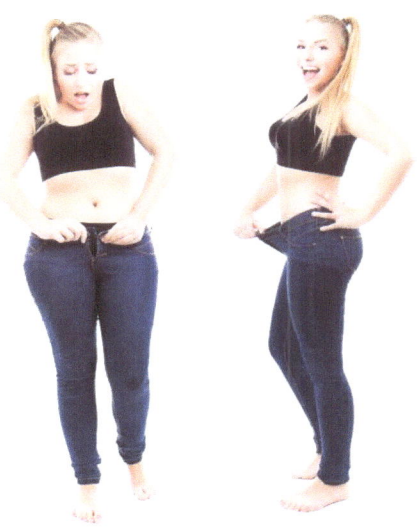

In trying out any diet, it is of utmost importance that you familiarize yourself with all the do's and don'ts that accompany it. For instance, you have to at least have an idea about the standard or recommended dietary guidelines of your chosen diet in order to achieve the results that you want. In this regard, I hope that you would be able to understand what the DASH Diet is all about and try at least some of the recipes listed in this book to meet your health needs and consequently lose those unwanted pounds.

As you have read all throughout this book, the DASH diet is one of the most natural and effective ways to live healthily and have a lower risk of developing serious illnesses. If you want to really have a lifestyle change and enjoy having a lower blood pressure and cholesterol, then I suggest that you start now. Remember that the DASH diet offers you a lot of benefits and following the tips and suggested meal plans in this book would definitely help you in getting started and remaining on this healthy path!

-- Emma Fisher

www.ingramcontent.com/pod-product-compliance
Lightning Source LLC
Chambersburg PA
CBHW050753290526
45792CB00008B/2158